THIS BOOK IS DEDICATED TO

The many residents of nursing homes
that I have had the pleasure to encounter.

Nursing Homes:
A Look Inside

CYNTHIA WIESNER BOWEN

TRAFFORD

• Canada • UK • Ireland • USA •

Note for Librarians: A cataloguing record for this book is available from Library and Archives
Canada at www.collectionscanada.ca/amicus/index-e.html
ISBN 1-4120-8086-X

Trafford's print shop runs on "green energy" from solar, wind and other environmentally-friendly power sources.

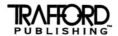
PUBLISHING™

Offices in Canada, USA, Ireland and UK

This book was published *on-demand* in cooperation with Trafford Publishing. On-demand
publishing is a unique process and service of making a book available for retail sale to the
public taking advantage of on-demand manufacturing and Internet marketing. On-demand
publishing includes promotions, retail sales, manufacturing, order fulfilment, accounting and
collecting royalties on behalf of the author.

Book sales for North America and international:
Trafford Publishing, 6E–2333 Government St.,
Victoria, BC v8t 4p4 CANADA
phone 250 383 6864 (toll-free 1 888 232 4444)
fax 250 383 6804; email to orders@trafford.com
Book sales in Europe:
Trafford Publishing (uk) Limited, 9 Park End Street, 2nd Floor
Oxford, UK ox1 1hh UNITED KINGDOM
phone 44 (0)1865 722 113 (local rate 0845 230 9601)
facsimile 44 (0)1865 722 868; info.uk@trafford.com
Order online at:
trafford.com/05-3084

10 9 8 7 6 5 4 3 2

ACKNOWLEDGEMENTS

For many years I have "threatened" to write a book about nursing homes as an outlet for my frustration regarding situations that seem to occur with frequency at the facilities where I have worked. My husband, Don, who is also a nurse shared my concerns for the treatment of the elderly and disabled. He encouraged me to educate the general public about long term care facilities with the hope that knowledge is the sword in the masses that will improve situations for the residents under our care. His compassion for those in nursing homes encouraged me in so many ways when I wanted to give up on the long and arduous task of writing a book.

My friend, Terri Woodley, always gives me insight to how the general public looks at a situation and often it is completely different from my perception as a nurse. She tolerantly listened to my concerns and gripes.

Thank the good Lord for the physicians like Dr. Chandra in this world. He frequently became our saving grace to make difficult work situations more tolerable. He could be counted on to respond quickly when called upon and to personally make rounds on his patients nearly every week. His obvious concern for the elderly and disabled was like a breath of fresh air in what at times seemed like a smothering, no win situation.

I am grateful to be able to find a publisher like Trafford. They were always willing to answer any questions I had and to guide me on my way.

The many residents I have had in the nursing homes I have worked in have always showed concern and appreciation for me and anything I did for them. Their words of encouragement was frequently the push I needed to make it through a long shift.

My appreciation for my parents grows with each passing day. Their memories of the past are cherished by me when they are shared and is part of why I prefer to work in nursing homes. The elderly represent the past and should be a reminder to us of how people have toiled and suffered to give us the comforts we enjoy today.

CONTENTS

CHAPTER 1

INTRODUCTION

I decided to write this book as an informational tool for the general public. Often while working, I wondered why residents and families came to a facility with preconceived misconceptions and were uninformed on even the basics of everyday life at a nursing home. I don't blame the families or residents when I have personally heard them given false or misleading information and promises by the social services department or admissions personnel regarding a resident's stay. I have even witnessed bullying by the staff to strongly urge residents on Medicare A to stay in the nursing home to at least the end of their twentieth 100 percent paid day, even when they felt they were well enough to go home and no longer qualified as needing skilled care.

I have worked in several western states and have found these problems to not be isolated incidences. I have also worked in facilities that have monitored their Medicare A residents and taken them off of Medicare services when they no longer qualified. Unfortunately, the opposite is true in others that have kept residents on Medicare A for the full 100 days with no real skilled services to speak of, just to keep the higher Medicare reimbursements coming to the facility.

Expectations of families and residents are often unfulfilled because of the misleading information given to them. This causes un-needed hostility between the residents/families and staff, often hindering a residents rehabilitation. Sometimes residents and families come in with the idea that the nursing homes now are like the ones they visited back 20, 30 or more years ago. Many are pleasantly surprised to find that unpleasant odors are at a minimum and quickly dissipate. Also, it quickly becomes apparent that the push is on toward rehabilitation and for the resident to do as much as possible for themselves. They are no longer treated as vegetables needing to be watered three times a day, but instead are encouraged to keep stimulated by increasing their independence.

Perceptions of residents may be different from that of their families and both may be different from the perceptions of the staff, even though they may all be looking at the same situation. Hopefully, this book will alleviate the distance between perceptions and draw everyone closer to do what is best for the wellbeing of the resident.

CHAPTER 2

PREADMISSION
TO A NURSING HOME

The dreaded day has finally arrived and you are approached to admit your loved one to a nursing home. It doesn't matter who first voiced the suggestion, a concerned friend, relative, family physician or nurse, the sinking feeling is the same. The connotation "nursing home" brings to surface feelings of giving up, almost like disposing of your relative just because they can no longer survive on their own. Immediate feelings of guilt and panic arise. No matter when the subject is broached, few are ready to take that step.

Questions like "couldn't they stay in the hospital longer?" or "isn't there more that could be done for them at the rehab center?", are commonly heard. Like many other things in our lives, this is also monetarily driven. Hospitals and rehab centers get Medicare and insurance reimbursement based on progress or need of skilled services. If an individual levels out or no longer makes progress with therapies and no longer requires acute care services, the pays source "dries up".

Acceptance to placement in a nursing home has as much to do with an individual's perception of long term care as it does with one's feelings of the need for placement. There can be a shock at the difference between the hospital and the nursing home initially. The type of care is now different, there is less availability of staff to meet your needs and anger that one's life is now totally changed, whether it is for a short period of time or for a long duration.

The majority of people faced with entering a nursing home feel a great loss of independence. Some feel relieved that they no longer have to worry about who will cut the lawn, do their laundry, take them to the doctor, etc. Many do not find the nursing home on their own and the burden of finding an appropriate placement is left to the family. The question now arises which facility is best? The answer to that question depends on what is important to you and what your family member's needs are.

Locality has a lot to do with one's choice of long term care facility. Is it near family? Is it near to your choice of medical facilities? Does your doctor have privileges there? The reasons for the nursing care can help you decide which one is best for you or your family member. Are they mainly being admitted for rehabilitation purposes, to increase strength and ability to care for themselves? Then, check around and inquire about rehab units in hospitals or extended care units. If they have a high drive for improvement in their ADL's (activities of daily living), such as dressing, walking, talking, cooking, toileting, etc, perhaps these places or a rehab center would be a better placement. They would have more intense therapies than at a long term care center where a therapist may only see them once or twice daily, for a limited time frame. If the person to be admitted is unable to participate in a rigorous therapy program, perhaps nursing home placement is the best choice for them at this time. Pushing for rehab depends a lot on the illness, accident or circumstance that put the person in this situation and their willingness to participate in rehab.

Facilities can be checked out on the internet, many have web sites available and now state survey results are also displayed in this manner. Yearly surveys are done by the state health departments to help maintain certain standards of care.

After the initial shock and realization that the time has come to move on, one ponders what nursing homes mean to them. Remembrances of walking into the front doors of a nursing home and being greeted by urine smells and the older generation leaning awkwardly in their wheelchairs, dressed in hospital gowns parked in the front lobby. A bare sterile environment and little reminiscent of a home atmosphere. Shudder after shudder, you try to shake off the remaining thoughts of your youthful experience and tramp grudgingly on over to the nearest nursing home on your list.

Manicured lawns and pleasant outdoor sitting areas greet you as you enter the parking lot and get out of your car. A deep breath and you pull open the front door, with the next breath you are a little shocked to discover that there is no urine odor!! Looking around the entryway you spot comfortable chairs, couches, plants and wall hangings that are pleasing to the eye. Appropriately dressed and well groomed individuals sitting upright and comfortably in their wheelchairs and other chairs scattered about the room. This alone can encourage you to venture farther into the building.

First impressions do mean a lot, so before talking to anyone regarding the admission process, take a walk around the building and look around. Observe how the staff interacts with the residents and with each other. Is it respectful? Pay particular attention to the touch and manner in which people speak. Beware of facilities where you don't see any management mingling with the staff and residents, especially those who don't even seem to know the resident's names. There are those who are in "charge" of our family member who don't even want to touch them or call them by name, is this who I want to take care of my family member? Is there an air of professionalism, yet a warm and friendly attitude among staff? Glance into resident rooms, check for neatness, cleanliness and the amount of space that each resident has to claim as their own. Is the nurses station enclosed to protect privacy, resident charts out of plain view and conversations between the staff or with the doctor less likely to be overheard by passersby.

Come at mealtimes to observe if the dining experience is a pleasant one. Can you hear yelling, babbling or shouting across the dining room of staff members? Are residents that are fed in full view of others, do they have food dribbling out of their mouths, etc. While walking around the building, did it appear to have proper heating or cooling? Things indicative of problems would be residents in dirty clothes, long/dirty fingernails, lingering foul odors, dirty floors, facility personnel discussing residents in common areas, certified nursing assistants rushing from room to room, empty activities calendar or one filled with nonspecific items. Look around the building for sitting areas for people to visit indoors and outside. Try coming in the evening to see if it is a quiet, restful environment, is the staff loud and can you hear the constant buzzing of call lights. Trust your instincts about the facility. Everything you have observed will help you form questions that you'll want to ask at the beginning of the admissions interview.

You are now ready to talk to someone after your walk through of the building. When you enter the nursing home, ask for the admissions director or the person in charge of admissions. Be prepared before you come. Bring any pertinent paperwork from home, hospital, doctor's office or other facility. Pertinent paperwork includes emergency contact phone numbers, powers of attorney for financial or healthcare, living wills, recent history and physical, Medicare/Medicaid or other insurance information/cards. Be prepared to sign a CPR (cardiopulmonary resuscitation) or DNR (do not resuscitate) paper. Whatever your family member wishes to have done if their heart stops suddenly or if they become terminally ill and wish no heroics. Most helpful would be if a living will is already filled out. We don't like to think about the unthinkable, but please have a mortuary picked out. Things at times do happen and it is even more difficult to answer these questions in times of duress, such as a sudden death.

Be sure to ask what the room charges are, what is covered by insurance and what you or your loved one will be responsible to pay. Find out what services are included in the monthly rate and what is considered to be additional costs. Are there transportation services available and is it an extra fee? Ask if the facility is Medicare and Medicaid certified. What level of care are they able to provide? If your loved one had a three night qualifying stay at a hospital and has Medicare, it may be that their first 20 days will be covered 100 percent by Medicare. This gives you a little breathing room to help establish monetary matters. Call any other insurance companies to find out if the policy has any nursing home benefits. If your family member lives on a fixed income, they may qualify for state assistance. The most popular assistance is the Medicaid program. Medicaid often takes three months to approve, but will pay back to the date of application, so it is important to start the application process as soon as possible. Some states have Medicaid programs run by the separate counties and provisions are different county to county. All the more reason to start the complicated process as soon as possible.

The admissions coordinator should be able to answer the majority of your questions, but beware of empty promises that cannot be upheld by the floor personnel due to unfeasibility. Many administrators, director of nurses and admission directors are often bonus driven and pushed by their company to increase their census. They may promise the moon and have no way of fulfilling that promise.

This would be the time to ask about staffing ratios for all shifts – the number of residents per staff (nurses and certified nurses assistants). Find out if there is a registered nurse on duty and do they have a nurse 24 hours a day. Does your physician have privileges there and how often does he visit residents at the facility? What are the routines of the facility, meal times, meal charges if you want to eat with them, smoking regulations, and what is the allowable furniture from home? Does the facility supply televisions and telephones in each room? Is there a therapy department and how often do they see residents? Which therapies are in the building – physical, occupational, speech or recreational therapists? How often are baths offered (twice a week is the most common)? Are leave of absences or overnight stays at home allowed? Can the facility handle IV's or intravenous therapy or would that require a readmission to the hospital? Are there safety devices in place such as an Alzheimer's unit, automatic door locks, etc. Many nursing homes strictly enforce the "right to fall" ideation to decrease the use of restraints. Restraints can be seen as lap buddies/seatbelts in wheelchairs, side rails for beds and even Geri-chairs that can tilt back or have lap tables.

Often services provided by the facility depends on whether you live in a big city or small town. For example, large cities will have portable x-ray services that come to the nursing home, whereas in a small town, the patient would have to be transported to the nearest hospital for an x-ray. Check to see if there is an availability of transportation, such as a facility van or escort service. Are the medications for the facility in house, from a local pharmacy or from a mail order pharmacy out of town? Can you pick your own pharmacy or must you use the facility's pharmacy? Availability of medications are often critical to the patient and delays, shortages or running out of medications are often distressful to them and can have health consequences. Ask how often your family doctor visits the facility and if he/she is readily available to problems that may arise. Available can mean by fax, phone, pager, on weekends and after hours.

What are visitation hours? Are pets and children allowed to visit? Be aware you may have to show proof of rabies vaccination for any animals brought into the facility. Ask if there are any facility pets or pet therapy. Many residents of long term care facilities look forward to seeing and petting any animal that comes into the facility. Inquire if there is a beauty/barber shop on the premises and what their prices are. Does the facility have any private areas to visit, make or receive phone calls? Is there a hospice room, where in case of severe illness or impending death where the resident can be moved into and where family may stay with them if they choose? What religious services are offered to the residents and how often are they held?

Check to see if the residents are allowed to keep and drive their own vehicles. Look around at the available parking, is it well maintained or is it snow packed in the winter and full of potholes.

What are the standard supplies provided by the nursing home – shampoo, lotion, toothpaste, toothbrush, razors, shaving cream, attends (adult diapers), combs, brushes, basins, water pitchers, wheelchairs, walkers, oxygen concentrators, oxygen tanks, etc. – or are there extra charges for these items? It is possible that many of these items can be provided by the family at a much lesser cost. Also ask if laundry services are provided or is it an extra fee.

If all or the majority of your questions are answered to your satisfaction and you wish to proceed with the admission, on we go to the next chapter and what to expect on admission day.

CHAPTER 3

ADMISSION DAY

Ideally admissions are more acceptable and have better outcomes for the resident and staff if they occur in the weekday morning. This allows for time for the orders to be received, medications to be ordered and received in a timely manner, the hoards of paperwork surrounding an admission to be discussed and completed, etc. Please remember to bring several days worth of clothing changes as the laundry turn around may be a couple of days. Pictures of family, wall hangings, a favorite bed spread, radio or television add to the homey look of a room. If there is room for a chair or dresser from home, please feel free to bring them. Cell phones are wonderful for places that do not provide a phone in each room. Please, please, please do not bring any expensive jewelry, family heirlooms, large amounts of cash, credit cards or checkbooks! Any sum of money can be locked in the business office for the resident to use on incidentals (ice cream, beauty shop, shopping, etc). Theft is less common in a nursing home due to mandatory background checks on their staff, but most facilities do have wanderers (confused residents who don't know who they are, where they are or what they are doing and may believe your belongings are theirs) and they also often cannot control visitor actions. As always, it is better to be safe than sorry.

The first day is also the best time to decide how one wishes to be addressed. Mr. Jones, Harry or a favorite nickname – whatever the resident is comfortable with is fine. Expect to see an inventory sheet that staff will record any belongings the resident brings into the facility. This helps in the event of lost articles along with placing the resident's name in black permanent marker on clothing or any other article belonging to the resident.

Generally on the first day or two, an injection is given in the forearm to test for exposure to tuberculosis. This is mandatory in long term care settings. Refusal to be tested can mean denial into the nursing home. If the resident has been previously tested positive or has had TB in the past, a chest x-ray is required to clear resident of active airway disease.

Medications brought from home may be checked by the nurse and sent back home if the resident is on Medicare A. If the resident is on private pay, medications can be used if they are in their original container with a pharmacy label and is allowed by facility policy. Some medications, particularly over the counter creams, eye drops, etc. may be allowed in the resident's room, although they may be required to be kept in a locked box.

Generally, on admission, it will be explained to the resident and family the meaning of full code, partial code and no code. Full code is requesting all medical assistance regardless of the circumstances. This requires staff to perform CPR to the fullest – chest compressions, artificial breathing, activation of 911, EMT response with IV medications and electrical shock to stimulate the heart. Partial code is wanting a full code in an emergency such as sudden cardiac arrest, but not when death is imminent due to a disease process such as cancer. No code is requesting that no resuscitative measure be taken in any instance. There are other considerations that can be discussed such as feeding tubes, blood products, artificial respirators (ventilators), etc. If a resident's health status changes for better or worse, the code status can be changed on request. The code status on admission is not set in stone for the rest of the resident's stay – circumstances change, as does everything in life. Everyone has the right to make a choice of what quality of life means to them versus just existing. Please make family members aware of the resident's wishes. If no power of attorney for healthcare has been chosen, now may be a good time to start the process. Choices are hard enough to make during duress and this would ease the burden greatly and also make your wishes known to all.

CHAPTER 4

AFTER DAY 1

One of the most common heard fallacies about nursing homes is that one can just lie there in bed and the staff can do everything for you. This is not true, particularly if you are in for rehabilitation and are working with therapies. Therapy will push you to go home and to do as much as you possibly can for yourself (use it or lose it theory). Be aware that medications and treatments may not be given to you at the exact time you took them at home. If a medication is ordered for 9:00 am, the nursing home generally has between 8:00 am and 10:00 am to give that medication or treatment. Understandably in an emergency situation, the time frame may be even greater.

Depending on the facility, a nurse may have twenty-five or more residents to give medicines to at 9:00 am and not everyone can receive theirs exactly at 9:00 am.

Meals are generally expected to be eaten in the dining room – choking does happen and one is more likely to receive help in a room full of people than sitting alone in your room. If you are used to taking a Motrin for aches and pains around 10:00 each morning, please ask for it. Many medications are ordered prn (as needed) and won't be routinely given unless requested by the resident.

Try as much as we would like, there are routines in the nursing homes that are hard to deviate from and have things run smoothly. One of the routines is to get everyone up out of bed in the morning and taken to breakfast. A resident's habit at home can be put into the resident's care plan, but generally state regulations prohibit getting anyone out of bed before 5:00 am. If the resident was a farmer and got out of bed at 4:00 am every morning of his life, exceptions can be made. If breakfast is served at 7:30 am, residents are to be out of bed at this time except for illnesses or special circumstance. Bedtimes are generally a little more lax, though many residents feel a need to be put to bed immediately after supper. A good rule of thumb to prevent digestion or reflux problems is that residents are to sit up for at least 45 minutes to 1 hour after completing a meal. Meals and menus are often set up by the corporate office, although some latitude is given to the individual facility. If you have a special request or certain dislikes, please feel free to let the dietary personnel know and they will let you know if substitutions are possible. I have heard that the hospital in Greeley, Colorado, even makes pureed food look appetizing by forming it to the original shapes and making designs on it. That is going the extra mile for your patients! Extra nutrients may be ordered if there are circumstances such as recent weight loss, malnutrition, poor appetite or to provide for wound healing. All residents are weighed every month and some every week to monitor weight loss/gain. A few residents need to be weighed daily to monitor for edema (fluid in the tissues causing swelling and weight gain). The dietary department can best answer questions regarding availability of substitutes during mealtimes, variety of foods and snacks. Snacks may be allowed in a resident's room if stored in a resealable bag or closed container. Facilities often face problems with ants, bugs and other creepy crawlies due to residents taking leftover food from meals back to their room with the intention of eating it later, but forget about it in their dresser drawers or closets. Many well intentioned family members or visitors bring food items for the resident that is often more than they can eat in one or two settings and then the food spoils, making it easy for bugs to move in. In many facilities, the majority of complaints one will hear will be about the food. It is very difficult to provide every meal for every resident's particular liking. Common statements heard are "the food is bland", "not enough variety", "it's not the way I like it" or "it's not the way I used to make it". Regardless how nutritious a meal is, it doesn't have any nutritional value at all if it isn't eaten.

Another major concern of residents is their room and who they are to share it with. Roommate compatibility being a huge issue. If one roommate is alert and has all their mental facilities, having the other roommate being confused, constantly babbling and rummaging through the first roommate's belongings is obviously not a good match. Frequent room changes can be very disruptive to the resident, especially confused residents who knowing where their room is may be the only constant thing they can remember. It is very disheartening to see a resident who has lived in one room for a period of time be moved to another room and be totally lost and unable to find their new room. Room changes should be discouraged in the long term care setting. Circumstances can arise that may make this necessary, but only after all other interventions have failed. Common problems are roommates who play their television sets or radios too loud, earplugs can easily solve this problem. Personal dislikes frequently arise, along with those who just don't want to share a room. Verbalizations like "I don't want her/him in MY room – move them somewhere else". Many facilities have adopted this rule – the one who complains, is the one who should move when another bed is available. Another common practice is that the facility can give a thirty day notice to any resident informing them of a room change. Room changes can be done before the thirty days if it is agreeable to the resident or power of attorney. In severe cases of noncompliance with the facility rules, residents may be given a thirty day notice to move out of the facility altogether. Generally this is due to uncontrollable behavioral problems, noncompliance with smoking regulations or being a danger to other residents.

Isolation of residents may become necessary if the resident develops a medical problem that can spread to others or they become so immune suppressed that they can easily become infected by other people. It then becomes an issue of health protection for the residents. Isolation may entail being put in a private room with signs on the door requesting all visitors check at the nurses station before entering the room. It may also involved being served meals on plastic dishes and eating with plastic silverware. Large red biohazard marked bags may be placed in the room and anyone entering the room may be required to wear gowns, gloves, masks, etc.. These are all protective devices and may be necessary depending on the particular situation and hopefully only for a short time.

Concerns regarding the bathroom is a big issue with many residents. It may not seem like a big deal to you or I, but having a roommate who is a bathroom hog when the dire need to use the restroom arises is a big deal to a resident. The number of residents to a bathroom can cause much anxiety and makes a huge difference if it is two or four.

Window placement often makes the world of difference to a nursing home resident. It is much more pleasant in a room to be able to sit and watch out a window, particularly if it has a good view. One of the best at providing this is the Banner Health facility in Torrington, Wyoming, where all residents have a window view due to their unique design.

Proximity of the room to the nurse's station is another consideration. When a resident requires a lot of care, they should be closer to the nurse's station and if they are fairly independent and are wanting a quieter environment, a room farther away from all the activity of the facility may be more desired.

All resident's rooms are equipped with call bells for the residents to be able to call for assist. They are not toys to be used to test the staff on how quickly they can respond or to see if it actually works. This takes away from someone who might actually need a staff member to assist them to the bathroom or calling because they are having chest pain. Even more unbelievable is the residents who put on their call light and immediately calls the facility on their private phones to tell the staff to answer their call light first. If this is the way a resident routinely summons staff, they need to be reeducated that they are taking personnel, who answered their phone call, away from their work to search for the appropriate staff to assist them and that their call light if often already answered by this time.

Appropriate clothing for the long term care facility depends on the resident. Rehabilitation oriented residents usually work best in loose fitting clothes, such as sweat suits, knits, etc. Residents who need to have staff dress them should not have tight fitting articles of clothing. Those who are bedridden do best with duster type dresses, sweat suits and slip on shoes or slippers. Usually high heeled shoes are not a good idea, they can cause a higher risk of falling. Age appropriate clothing should also be kept in mind – most elderly in nursing homes do not like to wear mini skirts or oversized jeans that ride half-way down their rear ends. If the facility does the resident's wash, clothing made of wool or 100 % cotton usually shrink and do not last through many washings at a facility. Due to the large amount of clothing that a facility washes, lost items do occur frequently, espe-cially unmarked items, socks and underwear. Clothing should be marked clearly with black permanent marker. Clothing tags can be used as long as they are sewn in tightly and don't fall off.

Care plans are an individual's plan of care throughout their stay at the nursing home. It is routinely updated every three months and more frequently in cases of changes of con-dition where the resident has a significant health decline or progress. Care plan meet-ings should be open to the resident and their family members to attend. Care plans include ADL care – if the resident requires special assist with dressing, toileting, ambulating, eating and should include use of any assistive devices, utensils, walkers, etc.. Care plans also outline the care a resident receives for each of their diagnoses and what medications they are on, along with any precautions the staff is taking to assure the safety of the resident. The care plan team generally consists of a nurse, dietary manager, social services director, activities director and often a certified nursing assistant who provides direct care to the resident. If you are not made aware when care plans are, ask the charge nurse and make them aware you would like to attend.

CHAPTER 5

VISITORS

Visitors are always welcome and most facilities do not have set visitation hours. Keep in mind the facility may lock their doors from sunset to sunrise for security reasons. There should be a doorbell next to the front door that can be answered to allow you access into the facility if the door is locked. Many residents have restrictions and if you are unsure, ask the nurse. These restrictions may include dietary or fluid restrictions, others may be restricted to bedrest for various reasons, still others may be on rehab programs requiring them to propel their wheelchairs and not have others push them. The staff does not make restrictions to be mean, but to prevent serious medical setbacks and further the progression of their rehabilitation. When the flu and cold seasons arrive, signs are frequently placed on the front door of the facility requesting any visitors that have symptoms of colds or flu to please delay their visits until the symptoms are gone. The elderly and medically compromised residents of a facility are very susceptible to viruses and they can have fatal consequences. Their immune systems are often weakened to the point that they just cannot fight even the flu.

Many facilities have residents who wander and wear alarms, a kindly act of holding a door open for a sweet looking gray haired lady may be unwittingly allowing an Alzheimer's patient to wander out onto a busy street.

The most common gift brought in by visitors is food. Staff can assist the visitor in deciding what type of food is appropriate for the resident and if sharing is allowed for roommates and tablemates in the dining room. Generally it is taboo for a visitor to feed a resident other than their family member for various reasons – for example, they may have a swallowing problem and may choke easily, even on water.

There are visitors, especially ones who visit frequently, that have a familiarity with the staff and especially around the Christmas holidays, wish to give gifts to the staff. Candy, baked goods, etc. are best to give. Money and expensive gifts are not allowed and it is against facility policies for any staff member to accept these items.

Conflicts that may exist between family members could be discussed with the social services director and should not involve staff members or other residents. The social services director will decide with the administrator if other staff members are to be involved in the situation. Please do not ask staff members to witness legal documents. The majority of facilities have policies against their staff acting as witnesses due to a possible conflict of interest. Frequently other residents are asked to witness another resident's signature, something that has questionable legality if the witnessing resident has a diagnosis of dementia, Alzheimer's or confusion. It is probably in everyone's best interest if all legal documents are prepared and dealt with before entering a nursing home.

Phone calls are welcomed for the residents. Inquire if the facility has a mobile phone that can be taken to a resident's room if they are in bed or carried to the dining room. If there is no mobile phone available, ask what time would be best to call the resident, when they will be out of bed, not in therapies and not at meals. Also inquire if phones have volume controls for those with hearing impairments. Don't call and demand a resident be woken up and gotten out of bed when you call, most people would not accept this behavior at their home nor is it socially acceptable at a nursing home.

Just because a person is admitted to a nursing home does not mean that they no longer wish to be included in family activities. It is always such a joy to see wedding parties in all their finery, stop in the nursing home so their family member who was unable to attend, can see them on their special day. Baptism parties that drop by so that the grandparent or great-grandparent can see the baby in their baptismal outfit or prom goers that hold off on their festivities and glide down the halls in their outfits to visit their family member are all occasions that give many residents joyous memories to recall for days to come.

Due to confidentiality protection of residents, if you are not a resident's medical power of attorney or close family member, information regarding a resident's medical condition cannot be disclosed to you by the staff. This is the hardest for people who live in a small town to understand why nursing home personnel won't tell them any information about their friends, neighbors and acquaintances.

For those who have not visited a nursing home in quite awhile, here's a bit of nursing home etiquette. Don't loudly announce (in front of visitors) to the staff "Mrs. Jones has wet all over herself, go clean her up" or "Mr. Jones smells horrible, take him to his room and check his pants". There is no quicker way to demolish a resident's dignity than words such as these. It is really demeaning to hear it frequently coming from the mouths of nursing home administrators, department heads and visitors who supposedly claim to be some of the greatest defenders of resident's rights. One can only imagine that the offenders believe all residents are either deaf or so confused that they have no understanding of the verbal language. Speak to others in a manner that you wish them to speak to you. The people who live in nursing homes are not invisible, don't talk about them or interrupt them as though they aren't there. It is considered rude outside the facility as well as within it's doors.

CHAPTER 6

ACTIVITIES / VOLUNTEERS

Activities are an important part of long term care facilities. Many residents look forward to certain events such as bingo, birthday parties, shopping, van rides, music programs, etc.. Activities such as these are often difficult without the help of volunteers. Volunteers perform all sorts of services. They read resident's mail to them, help write their letters and go shopping for those residents who are unable to leave the facility. Anyone can volunteer, from the very young to the elderly, male, female, it doesn't matter, all volunteers are welcome. Simple gestures such as offering to do sewing of buttons, mending clothes, making lap blankets or even visiting those who rarely get visitors is a wonderful way to volunteer.

Many community clubs and organizations volunteer their time and talent to long term care facilities. School groups perform plays, girl scout troops come in and sing songs, church groups hold services open to anyone who wishes to attend, all provide enjoyment to the residents who are unable to venture out and attend community activities on their own.

Special activities for residents are ones that have unique meaning to them and are the ones that remind them of days gone by, such as the parades they used to attend, festivals, operas, plays and even the hunting they used to do. Sharing of these activities often bring back some very fond memories for the resident and frequently they will share these times with you.

Since many residents are on fixed incomes, routine activities such as going to the barber or beauty shop now becomes a luxury they can no longer afford. Volunteers can perform haircuts, curl hair or even provide permanents for the cost of materials. It is amazing how good it makes someone feel just to have their hair fixed!

Facilities usually will have books or magazines for the residents to read, some of the real progressive nursing homes even offer their residents internet access! As many of you probably already know, time can pass quickly when one is surfing the web or reading e-mails.

Some facilities provide memorial services for residents who have passed away to give their facility friends a chance to attend a service without leaving the facility. It is a wonderful way to remember those who have left and gives those remaining a chance to mourn for them.

CHAPTER 7

MONEY MANAGEMENT / GIFTS

Money management for the nursing home resident is a cause of great concern for them. The majority have spent all their lives saving for their retirement only to discover that healthcare costs have eaten away their nest egg to the point that they now rely on Medicaid to pay for their nursing home costs and medical care. Medicaid/ social security residents are left with approximately fifty dollars a month to call their own. Yes, Medicaid provides them with a place to live, food , medicines and healthcare costs, but it does not provide for replacement clothing, perfume, cigarettes, candy, soda, replacement eyeglasses or dentures that become lost or broken, everyday items one is accustomed to using or having are all of a sudden too expensive to buy. Any of these items become wonderful gifts for birthdays, Christmas or just to bring when visiting the nursing home. If you need suggestions ask the certified nursing assistant or nurse caring for the resident, they may have plenty of ideas.

CHAPTER 8

HOSPITAL VERSUS
LONG TERM CARE

As baby boomers are now filling nursing homes, the majority of the population will know someone in a nursing home. As more people are associated with long term care facilities, the more the care provided will be in the public eye. As hard as it is to believe, sometimes the type of care is better in the nursing home than in the hospital. Residents who are immobile will at times return from a hospital stay with decubitus ulcers, Foley catheter placements and marks where restraints were used. Regulations for hospitals differ from nursing homes in several ways. Hospitals are free to use restraints, because of the acute circumstances that the patient is in that required the hospitalization, whereas in the nursing home the situation changes to chronic care and must be dealt with differently. In a hospital it is expected for a patient to be in bed, get meals served to them in bed and to be restrained if they become confused (as elderly often do in a strange environment or in response to some medications), to prevent them from getting out of bed, falling and pulling out tubes. This is also the reason bedsores can develop and why Foley catheters are inserted. In nursing homes the expectation is for the resident to get out of bed to prevent bedsores, to be toileted to prevent incontinency and they now have the right to fall rather than be restrained. The focus in nursing homes shifts to dealing with chronic illnesses and prevention of acute flare-ups or new problems.

The myth has been that only poor, lousy nurses or new graduates are best suited to work long term care, when in reality, the nursing home nurse needs a more extensive background due to the complexity and variety of illnesses in the elderly and incapacitated. The focus is not on the one thing that the person was admitted for in the hospital, but on a wide range of conditions.

The acuity or complexity of care for each resident doesn't count in the long term care center as it does in the hospital. The only reason for increasing staffing in the nursing home is the number of residents and not the amount of care they require. In other words, if there are fifty residents that are able to dress themselves, toilet themselves and walk independently, the staffing would be the same as if all fifty residents required total care, unable to dress themselves, were incontinent of bowel and bladder and needed to be lifted to a wheelchair. Doesn't seem right, does it? This is the way the majority of nursing homes are operated. When census is low in a facility, pressure comes from the corporate office or owners to accept any resident regardless of the amount of care they require or the hardship it may place on the staff and in turn on the other residents. Makes one wonder when there are more department heads and office staff working on any given day than there are nurses and certified nursing assistants who provide the actual hands on care of the resident. Questions arise such as: Are nursing homes over managed? (Too many chiefs and not enough workers).

This brings us to the duties of each department in the long term care facility. Someone not familiar with medical facilities often voice their concerns to the nearest or most available staff member and not to the person who can solve their problem.

Take for example the families that will ask nursing assistants for medical information and then turn around and ask a housekeeper to assist a resident to the bathroom. It is also inappropriate to make discharge arrangements with the office staff and try to get them to call the doctor for orders. In the next chapter we hope to clear up the question of who does what in the nursing home.

CHAPTER 9

NURSING HOME STAFF

We will start our exploration into the job descriptions of the nursing home staff with the laundry personnel. They are responsible for washing all personal clothing, bed linens, towels, any facility wash, etc. Any missing articles of clothing report to this person, because they are in the best position to locate the item. They hang up washed clothing in closets and put away undergarments in dresser drawers. It makes their job so much easier when personal items are clearly marked and they will be able to escort you to the location of items that were unmarked and unclaimed.

Housekeepers are responsible for the cleaning of residents rooms, offices, nurse's stations, public areas such as the dining rooms and restrooms. In many facilities they cannot clean up bodily fluids (blood, vomit, urine, sputum and feces). These wastes must first be cleaned up by the nursing staff with the appropriate cleansers and then the area can be washed by the housekeeping staff. Housekeeping, like laundry is not a twenty-four hour a day employment, so when they are not in the building, the nursing staff takes over.

Maintenance takes care of fixing, repairing, installing or maintaining the care of the building and equipment. Any large or complicated jobs are generally serviced by outside technicians, this would include computer and telephone lines. Many facilities will require that the maintenance personal be notified before anything can be hung on the walls in a resident's room or to run the cable line for a TV. The three previous jobs are supervised by the Environmental Services Director. This individual orders supplies for these departments, supervises the workers and handles the scheduling of their shifts.

The dietary personnel consists of the cooks, dietary aides, Dietary Manager and the Dietician. The cooks are responsible for cooking the meals per each resident's dietary order. Any deviation from the resident's ordered diet must be okayed by the nurse, Dietician, Dietary Manager, Speech Therapist or Doctor. If a resident is on a diabetic diet, the cook can only serve what is on the diabetic menu for the day. She/he must also only serve the food in the consistency that is ordered (ex. Pureed, mechanical soft, etc.). Dietary aides are responsible for setting the dining room tables, including any specialty utensils, cups, etc.. They are usually also the ones who serve the drinks to the residents per each residents dietary order – any substitutions must be approved by the staff mentioned earlier. If a resident is ordered to have only thickened liquids, this is what the dietary aide must serve. The Dietary Manager is in charge of supervising the dietary crew, ordering the food in the allowed budget and scheduling of his/her staff. If this person is not the Dietician, an outside Dietician is brought in to review diet orders, monitor weight gain/losses and make suggestions to the Doctor regarding supplements, nutritional labs (ex. Albumin levels) and diet changes.

The Activities Director may have an aide to assist them or may totally run the department with the help of volunteers. This is the person who will be able to tell you when birthday parties are, which days bingo is held, outings to go shopping or to the Senior Center, etc. They are also the one most likely to accept donations for bingo prizes, birthdays, craft items, etc.. Activities will post an activities calendar that lists the activities in the facility for the month. Sometimes an activity listed on the calendar is cancelled or not done. If this is a frequent occurrence voice your concern to the Activity Director as it is their responsibility to maintain so many activities a month.

The Social Services Director is the person who is in charge of problems, whether it's family issues or behavioral problems of residents. The SSD should be able to explain in detail each of the resident's rights.

An Admissions Director is the person to speak to before entering the nursing home and should be able to explain in detail what is expected of you and what you should expect from the facility. Often this position is given to either a nurse, business office person or social worker.

Business office personnel consists of a Payroll/Benefits Manager and a Business Office Manager. In larger facilities there may be a secretary or receptionist to direct you to the appropriate individual you need or to answer the phone. Any money matters, billing, insurance coverage, Medicare/Medicaid qualifications questions that you have should be directed to the Business Office Manager. If you wish to leave money for a resident's account for a resident to spend, it is usually left with the Payroll Manager, who will log it in and give you a receipt. Most facilities do not allow one person to handle all the money coming into and leaving the building.

The Medical Records Manager handles all the medical charts in the building. If copies of certain records are needed, this is the person to contact. Be aware that only the resident themselves and their healthcare power of attorney can request copies. Insurance companies, doctor's offices and other medical facilities at times will make requests, but must have permission from the resident or their healthcare power of attorney before any requests can be granted.

If there is a therapy department in the building, it could consist of Physical Therapists, Occupational Therapists, Speech Therapists and therapy aides. Any questions regarding therapy progress or decline should be directed here. They may or may not allow visitors to observe during therapy sessions. Often it is up to the individual therapist. If they believe that the resident is performing differently or poorly while being observed, the therapist will request to have no visitors during therapy time. Therapy billing may be separate from the facility billing. It may be billed to Medicare A, Medicare B, a supplemental insurance or to the resident if not covered by the insurances listed. Usually before any therapy is started on an individual not covered by insurance, the resident or their power of attorney is notified of the costs. Screenings by therapy are provided by the facility to determine if the resident could benefit from therapy.

The nursing staff consists of the Director of Nursing, Assistant Director of Nursing, Staff Development Coordinator, MDS nurse, Charge Nurse, Medication Nurse, Treatment Nurse/Wound Care Nurse, Infection Control Nurse, Certified Nursing Assistants and Restorative Nursing Assistants. The CNA'S or certified nursing assistants provide the majority of the hands on daily care of the residents. A CNA may be a male or a female. Acceptance of females doing personal cares is generally allowed by both male and female residents, but not so for the male nursing assistant. Many female residents will refuse to allow a male nursing assistant to assist them with showers, toileting, dressing, etc.. This often increases the workload for their female counterparts, who in turn will have to "pick up the slack". Hopefully, with the increasing numbers of male residents in nursing homes, this problem should soon even out and allow for a "trade" of work/residents assigned. This would allow for male and female nursing assistants to work together, increasing the safety factor for both the CNAs and residents. Injury from lifting is notably decreased when two people are doing the lifting instead of one, there is less chance for sexual or physical abuse and often aggressive residents are more cooperative when facing two CNAs instead of one. The nursing assistants are primarily responsible for the bathing, toileting, dressing, grooming, etc. of the residents. The restorative aides continue the therapy programs that were started by the therapists. They ambulate residents, perform range of motion exercises, continue dressing programs and provide restorative dining for those with eating difficulties. At some facilities they even monitor bowel and bladder programs. Large group exercise on activity calendars are run by activities and not by restorative. Restorative is for small groups and two different disciplines cannot take credit for one activity as some facilities try to claim.

Floor nurses consist of LPN's (Licensed Practical Nurses) and RN's (Registered Nurses). They often perform several different functions as Charge Nurse, Medication Nurse and Treatment Nurse. Some states allow Medication Aides to pass medicines to the residents. This is a certified nursing assistant with additional training in medication administration (usually 3-4 months). The Infection Control Nurse tracks antibiotic use in the building and the possible trends of exposure. The Wound Care Nurse measures the progress or worsening of wounds. She is often the one who makes suggestions to doctors regarding different methods of wound care, dressings, ointments, etc.. The Staff Development Coordinator (SDC) is in charge of all employee education in the building. This individual will schedule numerous inservices to keep the staff up to date on current medical procedures and reinforce the use of current practices. The SDC also tracks immunizations for both staff and residents. The MDS (Minimum Data Sheets) Nurse is in charge of filling out the resident information and assessment forms that are required by the state and federal government. She is usually the nurse who attends care plans and makes suggestions for changes to these plans of care. The Assistant Director of Nursing (ADON) assists the Director of Nursing with managing the nursing staff. She/ he will often be the one who makes the work schedule for the nurses and cnas. The Director of Nursing (DON,DNS) is the manager of all nursing staff. This individual attends all managerial meetings, disciplines the nursing staff, performs the hiring or firing of nursing staff. The DNS monitors the nursing department for the quality of care and to assure that all nursing staff are performing their duties assigned to them. As with the floor nurses, smaller facilities frequently combine the Infection Control Nurse, Wound Care Nurse, MDS, SDC, and ADON positions.

The Administrator or Executive Director is the overall manager of the building. They are ultimately responsible for the budget, staff and overall care of the residents. If your concerns are not met with any of the disciplines listed, bring your matter to the attention of this person. Be cautious of an administrator who continually voices that this is his/her building and not the resident's home. It creates doubt that this individual has the resident's best interests at heart. Also, if this person seems more concerned about the appearance of a building rather than resident's affairs, it is uncertain whether he/she is genuinely interested in the care of the residents.

The Medical Director is a doctor in charge of the medical services of the building. He/she ensures compliance with state/federal regulations regarding all medical issues. They educate doctors with facility privileges regarding their responsibilities and overseas the healthcare of the residents.

One person cannot run a whole facility, it takes a team. It is very difficult to manage a facility that operates twenty-four hours a day, seven day a week, fifty-two weeks a year. Nursing homes do not deal with objects, but with people and it is not an easy job to try to satisfy everyone. Many times things don't go like "clock work". Due to shift work and weekend coverage the likelihood of "call-ins" are high. The staff are like everyone else, family emergencies arise, illnesses, etc. happen and frequently it becomes a near impossibility to maintain the amount of people working everyday that is needed to provide adequate care. Facilities in larger cities have the advantage of calling in "pool staff" to fill the gaps, but in smaller towns there isn't that option on a daily basis. Job satisfaction can play a big role in absenteeism. Many facilities do nothing to motivate staff retention. There are no routine or menial merit raises, no cost of living raises and no retention bonuses. Complaints that managerial attention is directed mainly at "peripheral trimmings" or how a building looks, rather than how the residents and staff are taken care of. When there is no private bathroom, break room or smoking area for the staff, they are really unable to take a break that is uninterrupted, unless they leave the facility. Conflicts of interest with supervisory personnel, favoritism, staff supervising family members on an unprofessional level frequently causes undue stress to the employees and are often felt by the residents. Employees that are not disciplined for continually not doing their job sets a poor example for others (they didn't do their job and nothing happened – why should I make the extra effort to complete my work?). Sad, but often these stressors outweigh the benefit of helping people in need (residents) and lead to the loss of valuable employees. Whenever visiting the facility, look around, does the staff appear to be rushing around or as the new ideation puts it "challenged on the floor". If this is the case, it may mean that the facility does not have enough staff to meet the needs of their residents. Staff will be told not to mention when they are understaffed, but visitors and the residents themselves are not all blind, deaf or demented. When there are usually four Cnas providing care on a certain shift and all that are seen is two Cnas, it doesn't take a genius to figure out that the shift isn't adequately staffed. Many facilities run under the assumption that when extra help is needed, supervisors will leave their offices and help – it is an exceptional facility where this happens as a rule.

What is adequate staffing? Adequate staffing is what is needed to get the job done, providing safe and complete care of the residents. It should always be taken into consideration the amount of time required to provide suitable care. Take for example a reasonable amount of time required to get one resident out of bed should be at least fifteen minutes. This includes assisting them out of bed, wash their face, brush their teeth, help them dress, assist them to the toilet or clean them if they are incontinent, brush their hair, shave them, etc.. If Cnas are starting their shift at 6:00 am and breakfast starts at 7:30 am, then each of the Cnas should have six total care or assisted care residents to get up each morning. If each of the Cnas has twelve residents to get out of bed for breakfast, expect to see the telltale signs such as dirty dentures, hair not combed, eyes that are mattered with "sleep", disheveled clothing, body odors, etc. and meals not being served on time. Whether the staffing is adequate or not, the resident and family always have the option of hiring private duty nursing (Cna/nurse) to provide extra care of the resident. Private duty nursing care is in the employment of the resident or family and are not in the facility to supervise the staff.

There have been reports of unreasonable demands being made of the staff. Comments like "you will do my mother first" and demanding staff leave another resident to tend to their family member. Mind you, if the family member was in distress or had fallen, these requests are reasonable. Too frequently this is not the case. The staff does recognize that families just want the best care possible for their loved one, regardless if it out of guilt, helplessness or genuine worry for their welfare. Staff is paid by the facility and the resident/family pays the facility for their care. It is not uncommon to hear the old adage "I pay your salary and you will do everything I tell you". Yes, healthcare workers are there to assist you, but not become your private servant. Older adults place great value on living in their own home and often it is one they have lived in for decades. While at home they did everything in their daily lives a certain way and moving into a nursing home is a huge adjustment. When at all possible, attempts will be made to accommodate residents to have things done their way.

CHAPTER 10

RESIDENT RIGHTS

The prejudice or preconceived ideas that older adults and handicapped should not participate in certain physical or mental activities, that they are all alike, unproductive and resistant to change. This is all horse dodo. Many are stereotyped as not being able to speak for themselves, therefore have no rights and need to have everything done for them. This is why residents are given a list of their rights on admission to a nursing home. They do NOT lose their rights as an individual when entering a long term care facility! They retain the right to handle their own finances, they can refuse medications and treatments. They have the right to privacy, the right to vote, speak freely and any right they had before entering the nursing home. They are entitled to while in the nursing home, as long as they are in a sound mind, make decisions for themselves or if they are not in a sound mind, have their healthcare power of attorney make the decision for them. This is a common misconception, a healthcare power of attorney can only make decisions for the resident if they become incapacitated and unable to decide for themselves. Having a healthcare power of attorney does NOT mean that they can make decisions for a resident that can still speak for themselves.

Any decision that is made to refuse doctor's orders for medications or treatments must be an informed decision. The healthcare facility will inform the resident of the consequences of refusing, such as: refusal to bathe, the health risk and facility requirement may lead to discharge from the facility. The refusal of medication may lead to a decline in health status or the refusal to follow a diabetic diet may lead to hyperglycemic episode, stroke and death. Leaving the facility against medical advise may lead to denial of readmission, Medicare A's denial of payment of services and the cost of the long term stay will become the responsibility of the resident to pay. The right to date and have sexual relations with another person is also a right that cannot be denied as long as the other person is a consenting adult with intact mental capabilities. It will not be allowed for one resident to take advantage of another resident's confused state of mind.

All residents have the right to prepare advance directives regarding any medical decisions they want done if they become physically or mentally unable. They have the right to chose their own healthcare and financial power of attorneys. The resident has the right of privacy with phone calls and visitors. The right of privacy also includes the confidentiality of their medical condition and record.

Residents are ensured the freedom from any type of abuse.

It makes no difference whether it's mental, physical, sexual, verbal or emotional abuse. They are also to be free from restraints – physical or drug induced. Some facilities go as far as no side rails, even half rails that assist residents to reposition themselves.

Residents must respect other resident's rights, follow facility rules and give the facility accurate personal/medical information. If one feels that their resident rights have been violated and is not satisfied with the facility's response, they can notify the Ombudsman to intercede on their behalf. An Ombudsman is not associated with any nursing home and can mediate between the resident and facility. It is the Ombudsman job to investigate any infringement of the resident's rights. The phone number for the Ombudsman should be hanging on the wall in a prominent place in the facility. The resident council is a group of residents representing all the residents in the nursing home. Any resident is welcome at their meetings to express any concerns that they may have. Concerns are then passed on to the administration of the facility to resolve.

CHAPTER 11

FALLS

Falls are to be expected to be common place, especially right after admission to the nursing home. The resident is coming into an unfamiliar environment, recovering from an illness, are weak, perhaps disoriented from a recent medication change and are no longer confined by restraints of side rails, medications or other physical binders that were used in the hospital. When considering a resident's safety on admission, the nurse will assess for the inability of the resident to comprehend safety issues, their overestimation of their physical abilities or their lack of awareness of their obvious physical limitations. The nurse may then initiate the need for safety devices.

It may be as simple as a mat next to the bed to cushion any possible falls out of bed. The resident may also be placed in a low bed which is close to the floor to lessen the chance of injury and perhaps the use of positioning pillows are to be used. It is possible that a bed or chair alarm will be instituted. These alarms do not prevent falls, but can alert the staff that the resident is attempting to transfer themselves or that they have fallen and need immediate assist. There are all types of bells and alarms in a nursing home. There are call lights, bathroom/emergency lights, door alarms, bed/chair alarms, etc.. The staff needs to be aware of the different sounds and which require immediate attention. Other safety measures may be used to prevent or lessen the likelihood of a fall, such as moving the resident to a room closer to the nurse's station to hasten the response time.

The use of lifts to transfer residents can also reduce the number of falls. Resident run the increased risk of falls during transfer due to combative behavior or fear of falling and grabbing onto furniture/staff. Lifts can include a Hoyer lift that places a sling under the resident and a mechanical device lifts them to a wheelchair, commode chair or bed. There are also stand up lifts that assist the resident from a sitting position to a standing position and back to a sitting position. All falls are charted on the resident's medical record along with any injuries and notifications of family and doctor.

CHAPTER 12

BATHING

It is common for the elderly at home to do "spit" baths or washing oneself off with a washcloth, without actually entering a bath-tub or shower. This causes a problem in the nursing home where facility and state regula-tions require the resident to be totally bathed twice weekly. Frequent excuses heard are "it's too cold", "I'm too tired", "I washed off this morning" and "I already had a bath this week". Residents do have the right to refuse baths at times, but due to the health code agreement signed by the resident on admission, it is a nursing home regulation that if not followed may lead to dismissal from the nursing home if it becomes a frequent problem.

Refusing to bathe when offered may give up the chance to bathe until the next bath day. Bath days are assigned to provide everyone with the chance to bathe twice weekly, taking into account the number of staff per shift and the number of shower rooms available in the facility. There may be more flexibility with bath days and times when a facility has a bath aide. A bath aide is a Cna who does all the bathing in the facility and is not restricted by other duties.

CHAPTER 13

TYPES OF NURSING HOME RESIDENTS & FAMILIES

There is no longer one "type" of nursing home resident and hopefully gone are the days when family members take grandma for a drive and drop her off at the nursing home. Just as geriatric care is increasing in frequency and complexity due to expanded life spans, so is the care of the disabled younger generation growing. Younger people, even children are increasing in numbers in the long term care facilities. It may be due to accidents, disease or inability of family to care for them at home.

Caregivers have endless lists of responsibilities. They feed, bathe, shop, pay bills, do laundry, take care of the yard, do housework, drive to doctor's appointments and the list goes on. There are so many demands that many caregivers are inadequately prepared to handle the high stress and meet the demands of their own family if they are in a separate household. They or the person they are caring for may express frustration when they feel they have less control over the care in the nursing home. They may act out with frequent complaints, suspicion toward staff and even hostility. The staff can empathize with the family, but cannot provide special attention or privileges for one resident when it may take away from the care of other residents.

Do not be afraid to voice your concerns. There may be a middle ground that can be reached to ease the minds of all involved. Appropriately call attention to your concerns to the right person or persons. If you have a problem with something not being done or being done inadequately during the week, don't demand the weekend shifts to fix the problem. Chances are they have little control over another shift. Direct your displeasure to the Charge Nurse, Director of Nursing or Administrator. Requests can be made to the nursing assistants, but if not with satisfactory results, carry your concerns to the Charge Nurse. Keep in mind that this is a facility that is run by humans, taking care of humans and human error does occur. There has yet to be invented a perfect human being without the capability to make mistakes.

Another growing group in nursing homes are those being pushed out of psychiatric hospitals due to overcrowding. Unfortunately, this also increases the amount of behavior type problems witnessed and frightens many residents. It is very disturbing to see someone "lose control" by yelling, screaming, throwing things and suddenly striking out at others. No one wants to see their residents in danger and episodes such as these can be more controlled with medications, employee training and if needed discharge to a more appropriate facility.

Short stay residents are more common in facilities with rehab departments. Yes, today going to a nursing home does not necessarily mean one is sentenced for the rest of their natural life. Therapies can greatly increase the rate of resident discharges to home and once a resident is well enough to take care of themselves with minimal outside help, they are discharged from the facility. For many who stay at the nursing home, there is a sense of security that someone is close by to check on them, provide meals, assist them to the bathroom if needed and to be just a call bell ring away.

CHAPTER 14

DISCHARGES / LEAVE OF ABSENCES

The nursing home is not a prison and residents are allowed to go on leaves of absences (LOA's) to church, family functions, visits, out to eat and even overnight stays. Make arrangements ahead of time if the resident is leaving for an extended period of time. This gives the staff time to prepare medications, get authorization from insurance companies if needed, pack their bag, etc.. Discharges to home are a joyful and much anticipated event for many residents. Usually this occurs after therapy evaluates a resident's home for safety issues and releases the resident from therapy as able to perform well at home. A Doctor's order will be received, Home Health, Meals on Wheels and oxygen providers will all be notified if needed prior to the discharge. Everything possible will be done to try to make the discharge process a smooth one. The nurse will go over the discharge instructions including which medications that the resident will need to take at home, any special instructions from the doctor and when the next doctor's appointment should be. Please take home any medications from the facility if the facility's policy allows. Medicare, Medicaid, private insurance or you have already paid for them and if they are left, they will be thrown away. Medications are not cheap by any means. Transportation home is usually provided by the family, but under certain circumstances, it may be provided by the facility.

Another type of discharge is not so favorable and that is the discharge to the hospital. Generally this is done under emergency situations, the resident became seriously ill and it could not be managed at the nursing home. The EMS (Emergency Medical Services) or ambulance will be called for transport to the hospital. The EMTs will arrive, evaluate the resident and transport them to the hospital. Hopefully this will be done in a professional and respectful manner. Episodes of EMTs grudgingly coming to a nursing home for transports have been witnessed. Complaints heard by all, that they are wasting their time taking an elderly resident to the hospital. This behavior is shameful and should be stopped immediately by the nurse on duty and reported to the Emergency Department Supervisor.

Some residents have a poor response to hospitalizations, the invasive procedures, strange/new environments and whenever possible should be kept at the nursing home. Most nursing homes have the trained staff and equipment to do intravenous therapy and can draw blood for labs. More and more nursing homes are becoming an extension of the hospital and are for more skilled care instead of just "maintenance" care. The trend to reduce the mortality rates in the hospitals has and will send more critically ill to the nursing homes.

CHAPTER 15

COMMON ILLNESSES –
WHAT TO EXPECT

There are residents that will be more prone to decline, regardless of the care provided, but the push for rehabilitation is the focus of numerous nursing homes. Residents and families will voice that they really weren't informed of what to expect as an outcome of the condition they suffer. It is difficult to predict exact outcomes and it may all depend on the willingness of the resident to work with therapy.

One of the most common admissions is due to Cerebral Vascular Accident (CVA) or stroke. When a debilitating stroke occurs, it will leave one side of the body weak or paralyzed (the opposite side of the brain affected). Stroke victims may experience a loss of speech, but this does not mean a loss of sound mind. They may show anger suddenly, feel depressed, may laugh or cry easily or unexpectedly. The sooner therapy starts and continues with these residents, the better the outcome. Even if the mobility does not return to the affected side, they are taught alternative ways to transfer, dress themselves, etc.

Another familiar admitting diagnosis is a fractured hip. Rehab is successful even with those in their eighties and nineties. Fracture hips used to be a death sentence, but that is no longer true. If a resident is motivated and makes the effort with therapy, many of these residents can walk again.

Incontinence is a leading cause for long term care placement. It is a social as well as a hygiene problem. The causes can be due to multiple pregnancies, immobility, medications or another medical problem. It decreases one's socialization, causes embarrassment, increases the risk of falls and skin breakdown.

Incontinent products are available and should be used in the nursing home to help preserve the dignity of those with incontinence problems. Forgetfulness in the elderly may be a problem and they may just need reminders to go to the bathroom.

Medications, infection, dehydration and hypoxia (low oxygen levels) can be the cause of sudden confusion and with proper treatment can be resolved. Serious memory loss that requires admission to a long term care center includes forgetting recent occurrences where cues do not assist in recall and not remembering persons or places. When the person cannot follow written or spoken directions, they lose objects, find them but forgot it's purpose are signs of Alzheimer's Disease or Dementia and can increase the difficulty of caring for this person in a home setting.

Regardless of the reason for the nursing home admission, make sure the nursing home you choose is equipped to handle your loved one's unique problem.

CHAPTER 16

END OF LIFE

It has been said by the terminally ill that cures are sometimes worse than the disease itself. This is particularly true for the elderly and chronically ill, who often prefer a quality of life to the quantity of life. When a resident comes to term with imminent death, it is the facility's responsibility to provide humane care at the end of their life. Communication with the resident and family is of the utmost importance at this time. All questions should be answered as honestly as possible and details should be sorted out in preparation for the end. A Do Not Resuscitate or DNR should be signed and hopefully this was done much earlier. It is difficult for the health care proxies to do, since they tend to be more protective than the residents themselves. Remember to keep in mind the resident's wishes above all else. It is much easier on the Healthcare Power of Attorney if the resident spells out when to withhold or give treatment and what they want for hydration, nutrition and pain relief. It should also specify if there is to be any donation of organs or body tissue. CPR does not have a success rate for anyone dying with a terminal illness, it causes undo trauma to the resident and is devastating for the family to witness.

Hospice is generally the major provider of end of life care, particularly the last six months. If the facility does not have Hospice services, ask if the resident could be moved to a Comfort Care room. Comfort Care rooms allow for family members to stay with the resident, even over night if they so wish. It should be a private room, away from the noise of the nursing home daily activity and should provide a soothing atmosphere. Comfort for the resident is the main objective now. Pain in the elderly is often untreated or under-treated due to concerns about the effects of the medication or resident/family anxiety regarding addiction. Keep in mind that addiction is not an issue now and no one wishes for the resident to suffer needlessly. The nurses will make all attempts to give pain medications as ordered to promote comfort for those in their final days.

CHAPTER 17

WHY DO NURSING HOMES ALWAYS SEEM TO BE SHORT OF HELP

Working in a facility that operates twenty-four hours a day, every day of the year, means working different shifts, weekends and holidays. The majority of workers are women, who are the primary caregiver of sick children and have spouses or significant others who oppose the shift work. Nursing homes do have volatile residents with histories of violence, alcoholism, psychotic diagnoses and dementia. It may seem unbelievable, but many people believe that if you work in a nursing home it is an accepted part of the job to be hit, kicked, bit and slapped. What other job would allow this to happen to their employees? Just as the residents are protected against harassments (verbal slurs, unwanted sexual comments, visual conduct such as gestures, physical conduct like assault and unwanted touching), so are the nursing home employees. Or so one would like to think. It creates an intimidating, hostile and offensive work environment that is frequently poorly monitored. Many episodes are underreported due to the lack of support from administration. Fairly common place are treatment from a select few residents that include cursing, racial slurs and threats such as "I'll get you fired". Is it any wonder that many facilities have a high turn over rate. When episodes are reported, they are shooed away with responses like "well you know they have Alzheimer's" or "the state won't allow us to have anyone else on psychotropic medicines".

When the workload is overwhelming, it also increases the risk of injury to the staff member, particularly back injuries from the extra lifting and strain. Inadequate employee acquisition, supervision and lack of retention practices also lead to a high turnover rate. Pay raises if given are seen as a pittance and viewed as insulting. Many facilities do not have cost of living raises. Nurses and Cnas feel that their experience is not valued and when they stay their salaries plateau. New employees often make the same wage as those with years of service to the facility. There is a huge liability of working in an environment of high responsibility, where workloads are increasing due to the growing numbers of severely ill and obese residents. As everywhere else government regulations are growing along with the mounds of paperwork and pressure from administration to reduce time on the clock.

Perceptions of the clinical nurse and administration is increasing in difference every day. Nurses can easily see the relationship between the level of staffing and the quality of care. It often puts them at odds with management and increases the job related stress.

CHAPTER 18

STATE SURVEY TEAMS

Nursing homes are surveyed annually as soon as nine months or as late as fifteen months from their previous survey. The certification from the previous survey should be displayed on the wall near the front of the building. Surveyors may make focused visits to the facility or investigate complaints at any time. They will usually focus their survey on risk factors in the facility. These risk factors include behavioral symptoms, bowel/bladder incontinence, antipsychotic medication use and pressure ulcers. During their visit they will also look at the direct care provided for residents and how quickly a resident in need receives assist. Surveyors may look at the proximity of resident's room to the nurse's station – some states have a limitation on how far the furthermost room can be to the closest nurse's station. They are available to talk with residents, families and staff regarding any concerns they may have pertaining to the care in the facility. In addition, they make sure that each resident and staff member is checked for TB (tuberculosis) and that vaccinations for flu/pneumonia are provided for residents unless medically contraindicated. Influenza shots are given every fall and the pneumonia vaccine given once past age 65. Staff in facilities with problems generally welcome the yearly survey and see it as a chance for improvement, since nursing homes must meet the survey teams demands to fix problem areas.

CHAPTER 19

INSURANCES –
MEDICARE, MEDICAID AND
PRIVATE INSURANCES

The majority of care provided in nursing homes is paid for by the government in the form of either Medicare or Medicaid. Medicare A is the insurance most elderly and disabled will have as their primary insurance after a qualifying three night stay at a hospital. Medicare A is very therapy driven. In other words, as long as the resident is making gains in therapy Medicare A will continue to pay for their stay (100% the first 20 days, 80% the next 80 days). The other primary things that will continue Medicare payment during this time is any medical complication, the prevention of deterioration, observation/assessment of risk factors, safety issues and hopeful return to prior level of function.

Medicaid is the insurance for long term or maintenance care for those who meet the qualifications. It pays for the resident's stay including room cost, medications and all supplies/services provided by the facility for a set amount each month. It may also cover the 20% that Medicare A does not in the last 80 days of a Medicare A stay. Private pay or private insurance will need to pay for everything separately, unless you are able to negotiate a set monthly rate with supplies and services included. Depending on what insurance policy you have will determine what is covered and what is not. Bring the policy to the Business Office Manager and they will help you sort it out.

CHAPTER 20

MISCELLANEOUS

Miscellaneous covers a wide range of topics, so this chapter may seem a little hodge podge. One may hear the term MDS used in the facility and wonder what it is. The Minimum Data Set or MDS is an assessment that determines whether quality of care was provided and the outcome of that care. It is a comprehensive assessment of each resident's status. When the MDS is completed it is sent electronically to the state Department of Health and can be what they base their yearly surveys on.

Each facility tries to encourage physical and mental stimulation because of the belief "use it or lose it". Most nursing homes are open to any ideas as activities for the residents. Popular interventions have been Trivia games and Walk to Dine programs.

Alcohol use is allowed in the nursing home if not medically contraindicated. Appropriate occasions would be holidays, wedding anniversaries, New Year's Eve, cultural dining, etc. This and any other religious and cultural considerations should be brought to the attention of the staff so they may be made aware of special observances for the resident. Please alert the staff to any fasting or abstinences that the resident may practice.

The United States is known for being a melting pot and this is becoming especially more evident in the nursing home population. More workers have foreign accents (what is foreign anyway depends on where you live) and language barriers. Communication is a huge concern, but is workable with gestures, simple words, language dictionaries, etc. which can ease the burden. Some of the hardest working long term care workers have started their lives outside of U.S. borders. A few of these have worked in healthcare in their original countries and need to be acclimatized or educated to the healthcare practices in the United States. What may have been acceptable in their country is not tolerated here. All facilities maintain orientation programs and abuse awareness programs.

Residents have a natural concern for their roommates, staff and other residents. Due to confidentiality only a limited amount of information can be passed along regarding another resident's condition, recent hospitalization, falls or death. It's helpful if regular staff tells the residents when they are going on vacation, leaves of absences and when they will be returning. It may be a little thing, but it eases a resident's mind.

The facility has health and safety programs that need to be routinely practiced. A couple of these are fire and evacuation drills. Residents and families need to be aware of fire alarms and cooperate with the drill. It may be necessary to move to a "safe" area and the door will have to be closed to the room. Nursing home evacuation policy will first evacuate the ambulatory residents (those who can walk), next will be wheelchair residents and last will be those that are bedridden. It is done this way in an emergency to save as many people as possible.

Most residents do not discuss their expectations of their doctor prior to the nursing home admission. The majority assume their doctor will visit them like they did at the hospital and are sorely disappointed when this doesn't happen. Talk with your physician and ask how often he/she will see you in the nursing home and ask how available he/she is to the nursing home staff should you develop a problem. Be sure to find out if your doctor has privileges at the nursing home you choose or you may be shopping for a new physician as well.

Medical advances are happening all the time and some things are hard for the resident to understand. In previous times, residents were accustomed to doctors prescribing them antibiotics for colds or the flu, nowa-days no antibiotics are given in these situa-tions. Medications are now decreased to a minimal number to prevent interactions with other medications. The nursing home staff as-sists the doctor with curing if possible, disease management, assisting with decision making, coordinating care with all involved, symptom control, optimizing quality of life and assist-ing with end of life care. Maybe the prestige of nursing in a hospital isn't there, but the self fulfillment of helping others who really need it is.

The nursing home decision can be a heart wrenching one and hopefully this book pro-vides one with a little more knowledge re-garding long term care.

ABOUT THE AUTHOR

Cynthia Wiesner Bowen was born in West Bend, Wisconsin, one of eight children to Jacob and Patricia Wiesner. Never really having much contact with nursing homes until entering nursing school in Wyoming in 1978. Beginning a nursing career as a Licensed Practical Nurse and received a Bachelors Degree of Science in Nursing in1988. Traveled and worked as a nurse in several western states, many times in nursing homes. She is married to Donnie Bowen, has 3 children – Katherine, Jonathan and Rebecca, 3 step-children – Donnie Ray, Susan and Donald Lee and 6 grandchildren – John, Amelia, Steven Clay, Kielee, Isaiah and Kambria.

Printed in the United Kingdom by
Lightning Source UK Ltd., Milton Keynes
138999UK00001B/42/A